MILLENNIAL-FRIENDLY RECIPES

Quick And Tasty Recipes For Weight Management

MICHELLE HAUGER

MILLENNIAL-FRIENDLY RECIPES

Introduction

Amidst the whirlwind of our contemporary world, time is a precious commodity for the vibrant generation of today. Balancing demanding professions, bustling social circles, and many responsibilities, millennials find themselves immersed in a constant dance of commitments. In the midst of this bustling existence, the imperative to nurture their bodies and sustain a healthy weight can often get overlooked. Nevertheless, precisely within these hectic moments, the utmost importance of swift and uncomplicated recipes, meticulously curated to complement their fast-paced lifestyles, comes to the forefront.

Maintaining a healthy weight cannot be overstated in a society increasingly focused on well-being and self-care. Weight management impacts physical health and is pivotal in mental and emotional well-being. For millennials, who find themselves at the forefront of a health-conscious era, striking the right balance between fitness and busy schedules is a delicate art.

The goals of weight management are as diverse as the individuals pursuing them. Some people seek to embrace their natural body shape and maintain a stable weight, exuding confidence in their skin. Others aspire to embark on a weight gain journey to achieve a healthier and more robust physique. Simultaneously, there are those driven by the ambition of weight loss, endeavoring to shed unwanted pounds and unlock the full potential of their well-being.

Amidst these varying aspirations, the common thread that unites millennials is their need for culinary solutions that align with their dynamic lifestyles. Quick and easy recipes act as a beacon of hope in the whirlwind of chaotic schedules, offering a lifeline to those yearning for nourishment without sacrificing time. These recipes are an empowering toolkit, enabling millennials to take charge of their health journey on their terms without compromising taste or nutrition.

Yet, the pursuit of a healthy weight should never be at the expense of flavor or satisfaction. The journey towards a well-nourished body need not be monotonous, filled with bland and uninspiring meals. Instead, it can be a compelling exploration of creativity in the kitchen, a delightful fusion of flavors and ingredients that cater to individual tastes.

With this in mind, the need for delicious and nutritious recipes that cater to the goals of both weight gain and weight loss becomes evident. A culinary repertoire that celebrates the vibrant hues of fruits and vegetables, the subtle balance of proteins and grains, and the enticing aromas of herbs and spices is the cornerstone of a sustainable and enjoyable health journey.

In this culinary adventure, taste, and nutrition become steadfast companions. Quick recipes incorporating abundant fruits, vegetables, whole grains, and lean proteins become the palette for millennials to paint their healthy future. Whether it's a refreshing and energy-boosting smoothie bowl to kickstart the day or a savory and wholesome grain bowl to refuel after a busy afternoon, these recipes become the building blocks of a nourishing lifestyle.

As people embrace the significance of maintaining a healthy weight and embark on their journeys, quick and easy recipes become their allies in the pursuit of well-being. These recipes are more than just culinary instructions; they represent a mindset, a way of life that champions self-care and self-discovery. In this world of delectable possibilities, individuals can savor the joys of nourishment without compromising on their busy schedules or diverse aspirations. It is a celebration of taste and health. This harmonious symphony resonates with the heartbeats of millennials seeking to embrace life to the fullest, one delectable and nutritious bite at a time.

SECTION ONE: MILLENNIAL RECIPES

In the fast-paced and digitally connected world of millennials, food has evolved beyond mere sustenance; it has become an art form, a means of self-expression, and a celebration of diverse cultures. As a generation known for its adventurous spirit and innovative approach to life, millennials have redefined the culinary landscape, infusing traditional recipes with modern twists and pushing the boundaries of flavor combinations.

From vibrant and Instagram-worthy smoothie bowls to delectable avocado toast variations, and quick and nutritious one-pot meals, millennial recipes cater to the busy schedules and adventurous palates of this tech-savvy generation. Embracing the principles of convenience, health-consciousness, and sustainability, these recipes showcase a harmonious blend of flavors, textures, and colors that entice both the eyes and the taste buds.

Here are some Millennial Recipes to satisfy the modern generation's taste for innovative and wholesome meals:

1. Acai Berry Smoothie Bowl

Ingredients:

- One frozen banana
- 1/2 cup mixed frozen berries (blueberries, strawberries, raspberries)
- One pack of frozen acai puree
- 1/2 cup almond milk (or any preferred milk)
- Two tablespoons granola
- Fresh berries (for topping)
- Sliced banana (for topping)

- Chia seeds (for topping)
- Shredded coconut (for topping)

Instructions:

1. Combine the frozen banana, frozen mixed berries, acai puree, and almond milk in a blender.
2. Blend until you achieve a smooth and thick consistency.
3. Pour the acai berry smoothie into a bowl.
4. Top the smoothie bowl with granola, fresh berries, sliced banana, chia seeds, and shredded coconut.
5. Savor the vibrant colors and nourishing flavors of this invigorating acai berry smoothie bowl, perfect for a nutritious breakfast or a midday pick-me-up.

2. Loaded Avocado Toast with Poached Egg

Ingredients:

- Two slices of whole-grain bread
- One ripe avocado
- One tablespoon of lemon juice
- Salt and pepper to taste
- Two large eggs
- Baby spinach leaves
- Cherry tomatoes, halved
- Red pepper flakes (optional, for extra kick)

Instructions:

1. Toast the slices of whole-grain bread until golden and crispy.
2. Mash the ripe avocado with lemon juice, salt, and pepper in a bowl.
3. Spread the avocado mixture generously on the toasted bread slices.
4. Gently crack the eggs and poach them in a pot of simmering water until the whites are set but the yolks are still runny.

5. Place the poached eggs on top of the avocado toast.

6. If you like, add some red pepper flakes, cherry tomatoes that have been cut in half, and baby spinach leaves as a garnish.

7. Indulge in this loaded avocado toast with a perfect balance of creaminess, protein, and a burst of flavors.

3. One-Pot Lemon Herb Chicken and Quinoa

Ingredients

- One tablespoon of olive oil
- Four boneless, skinless chicken breasts
- 1 cup quinoa, rinsed
- 2 cups chicken broth
- One lemon, zested and juiced
- Two cloves garlic, minced
- One teaspoon of dried thyme
- One teaspoon of dried rosemary
- Salt and pepper to taste
- Fresh parsley for garnish

Instructions:

1. In a big skillet or pot, heat the olive oil to medium-high temperature.

2. Salt and season the chicken breasts before searing them until both sides are golden brown. Take out and place aside.

3. Add the chopped garlic to the skillet and cook until pleasant to the taste, about a minute.

4. Add the rinsed quinoa, chicken broth, lemon zest, lemon juice, dried thyme, and rosemary to the skillet. Stir to combine.

5. Place the seared chicken breasts on top of the quinoa mixture.

6. Cover and let it simmer on low heat for about 15-20 minutes or until the quinoa is cooked and the chicken is tender and cooked through.

7. Garnish with fresh parsley and serve this flavorful one-pot lemon herb chicken and quinoa dish that's satisfying and time-efficient.

4. Spicy Sriracha Tofu Stir-Fry

Ingredients:

- One block of extra-firm tofu cubed
- Two tablespoons cornstarch
- Two tablespoons of soy sauce
- One tablespoon of sesame oil
- Two tablespoons sriracha sauce (adjust to taste)
- One spoonful of honey (or agave syrup for a vegan alternative)
- One tablespoon of vegetable oil
- One red bell pepper, thinly sliced
- One cup of broccoli florets
- One cup of snap peas
- Two cloves garlic, minced
- Cooked rice for serving

Instructions:

1. In a bowl, toss the cubed tofu with cornstarch until evenly coated.

2. Mix the soy sauce, sesame oil, sriracha sauce, and honey separately.

3. In a big skillet, heat the vegetable oil over medium-high heat.

4. Add the coated tofu cubes and cook until crispy and browned on all sides. Remove and set aside.

5. Add the minced garlic, sliced red bell pepper, broccoli florets, and snap peas in the same skillet. Stir-fry for a few minutes until the vegetables are tender-crisp.

6. Return the cooked tofu to the skillet with the vegetables, and then cover with the sriracha sauce mixture. Stir everything together, then heat for one more minute to coat everything in sauce.

7. Serve the spicy sriracha tofu stir-fry over cooked rice for a satisfying and flavorful meal that packs a punch.

5. Roasted Veggie and Quinoa Buddha Bowl

Ingredients:

- 1 cup cooked quinoa
- One sweet potato, diced
- 1 cup broccoli florets
- 1 cup cherry tomatoes
- 1 cup chickpeas, drained and rinsed
- Two tablespoons of olive oil
- One teaspoon of smoked paprika
- One teaspoon of ground cumin
- Salt and pepper to taste
- Lemon tahini dressing for drizzling
- Fresh parsley or cilantro for garnish

Instructions:

1. Set the oven temperature to 425°F (220°C).

2. Combine the diced sweet potatoes, broccoli florets, cherry tomatoes, and chickpeas in a large bowl with olive oil, smoked paprika, cumin, salt, and pepper.

3. Spread the seasoned vegetables and chickpeas on a baking sheet in a single layer.

4. In the oven, roast the vegetables until tender and lightly caramelized.
5. In a bowl, arrange the chickpeas, roasted vegetables, and cooked quinoa.
6. Drizzle with lemon tahini dressing and garnish with fresh parsley or cilantro.
7. This roasted veggie and quinoa Buddha bowl is a hearty and nutrient-packed meal that delights the senses and satisfies your hunger.

6. Vegan BBQ Jackfruit Tacos

Ingredients:

- One can of young green jackfruit, drained and rinsed
- 1/2 cup BBQ sauce
- One tablespoon of olive oil
- 1/2 red onion, thinly sliced
- 1 cup shredded purple cabbage
- 1/4 cup chopped fresh cilantro
- One lime, juiced
- Corn tortillas
- Avocado slices for garnish

Instructions:

1. Add the jackfruit to a skillet with the olive oil already heated over medium heat.
2. Once cooked and slightly browned, shred the jackfruit with a fork.
3. Stir in the BBQ sauce and let it simmer for a few minutes until well coated.
4. Mix the shredded purple cabbage, red onion, cilantro, and lime juice to make a slaw.
5. Warm the corn tortillas and fill them with the BBQ jackfruit and slaw.

6. Garnish with avocado slices and serve these delicious, vegan-friendly BBQ jackfruit tacos.

7. Mediterranean Chickpea Buddha Bowl

Ingredients:

- 1 cup cooked quinoa
- One can of chickpeas, drained and rinsed
- 1 cup cherry tomatoes, halved
- Diced cucumber
- About 1/4 Cup pitted and sliced Kalamata olives
- 1/4 cup crumbled feta cheese (or dairy-free alternative)
- Two tablespoons extra-virgin olive oil
- One tablespoon of balsamic vinegar
- One teaspoon of dried oregano
- Salt and pepper to taste
- Fresh parsley for garnish

Instructions:

1. In a bowl, mix cooked quinoa, chickpeas, cherry tomatoes, cucumber, Kalamata olives, and crumbled feta cheese.
2. To make the dressing, whisk together the olive oil, balsamic vinegar, dried oregano, salt, and pepper in a separate bowl.
3. Drizzle the dressing over the quinoa and chickpea mixture and toss until well-coated.
4. Garnish with fresh parsley and enjoy this Mediterranean-inspired chickpea Buddha bowl, packed with vibrant flavors and nourishing ingredients.

8. Cauliflower Rice Sushi Rolls

Ingredients:

- One head cauliflower, riced
- Two tablespoons of rice vinegar
- One tablespoon sugar
- One teaspoon salt
- Nori seaweed sheets
- Avocado slices
- Cucumber strips
- Carrot strips
- Cooked crab or smoked salmon (optional, for non-vegan version)
- Soy sauce and wasabi for serving

Instructions:

1. Combine the riced cauliflower, rice vinegar, sugar, and salt in a bowl.
2. Lay a sheet of nori seaweed on a bamboo sushi mat or a clean surface.
3. Spread an even layer of cauliflower rice on the nori, leaving a small space at the top.
4. Arrange avocado slices, cucumber strips, carrot strips, and cooked crab or smoked salmon (if used) on the cauliflower rice.
5. Carefully roll the nori into a sushi roll, using the bamboo mat to help create a tight roll.
6. Slice the sushi roll into bite-sized pieces and serve with soy sauce and wasabi.

9. Peanut Butter Chocolate Protein Smoothie

Ingredients:

- One ripe banana
- Two tablespoons of peanut butter

- One tablespoon of cocoa powder
- One cup of almond milk (or any preferred milk)
- One scoop of chocolate protein powder
- One tablespoon of chia seeds
- One tablespoon honey (optional for added sweetness)
- Ice cubes (optional for a chilled smoothie)

Instructions:

1. Blend the ripe banana, peanut butter, cocoa powder, almond milk, chocolate protein powder, chia seeds, and honey (if using) in a blender.
2. Blend until smooth and creamy.
3. Add ice cubes and blend again for a chilled smoothie if desired.
4. Pour the peanut butter chocolate protein smoothie into a glass and enjoy this indulgent yet nutritious treat.

10. Vegan Cauliflower Buffalo Wings

Ingredients:

- One head of cauliflower, cut into florets
- One cup of all-purpose flour (or gluten-free flour)
- A cup of unsweetened almond milk (or your chosen plant-based milk)
- One teaspoon of garlic powder
- One teaspoon of onion powder
- One teaspoon paprika
- Salt and pepper to taste
- 1 cup buffalo sauce (store-bought or homemade)
- Vegan ranch dressing for dipping

Instructions:

1. Wrap a baking sheet with parchment paper, then heat the oven to 425°F (220 degrees Celsius).

2. To make the batter, whisk the flour, almond milk, paprika, onion, garlic, and seasoning powders.
3. Place the batter-coated cauliflower florets on the preheated baking sheet after dipping each one into it.
4. Bake the cauliflower florets for 25-30 minutes or until crispy and golden brown.
5. Toss the baked cauliflower florets with buffalo sauce until well coated in a separate bowl.
6. Serve the vegan cauliflower Buffalo wings with vegan ranch dressing for a delicious and plant-based twist on a classic favorite.

Millennial recipes embrace culinary creativity and infuse traditional dishes with a modern twist. These recipes showcase a harmonious blend of flavors, textures, and colors, catering to the modern generation's adventurous palates and busy schedules. Also, they provide a delightful dining experience while supporting a healthy and balanced lifestyle. Enjoy the culinary journey of millennial recipes as you explore new tastes and culinary horizons!

SECTION 2: RECIPES FOR WEIGHT GAIN

Welcome to the world of nourishing and delicious recipes to support your healthy weight gain journey. Whether you want to add muscle mass, boost energy levels, or achieve a well-balanced physique, these recipes cater to your needs.

In a society that often focuses on weight loss, we understand the unique challenges faced by those striving to gain weight healthily and sustainably. To assist you in achieving your weight gain objectives without sacrificing taste or nutrition, our collection of recipes attempts to offer a variety of delectable and nutrient-rich solutions.

From energizing breakfasts to satisfying lunches and dinners, each recipe is carefully crafted to incorporate essential macronutrients and vitamins, promoting optimal health and well-being. Embrace the joy of culinary exploration as we guide you through a diverse selection of meals, snacks, and smoothies that nourish your body and inspire your taste buds.

So, join us on this delectable journey, where every bite is a step closer to achieving your weight gain aspirations. Let's embark together on a path of nourishment and self-discovery, unlocking the potential for a healthier and happier you.

Energizing Breakfasts

Discover a delightful array of healthy recipes that promote weight gain in a wholesome and nourishing way. These dishes are carefully crafted to provide the essential nutrients and calories needed to support your weight gain goals while keeping your well-being in mind. From energizing smoothie bowls bursting with goodness to satisfying avocado toast variations that delight the taste buds, this section is a treasure trove of delicious options to help you gain weight in a healthy and balanced manner. As you relish each bite, embrace the journey of nourishment and vitality, knowing that you are moving toward a healthier and happier version of yourself.

1. Vitality Berry Blast Smoothie Bowl

Ingredients:

- 1 cup mixed berries (strawberries, blueberries, raspberries)
- One ripe banana
- 1/2 cup Greek yogurt
- One tablespoon of almond butter
- One tablespoon of chia seeds
- One tablespoon honey
- 1/4 cup granola
- Sliced almonds and fresh berries for topping

Instructions:

- Combine mixed berries, ripe bananas, Greek yogurt, almond butter, chia seeds, and honey in a blender. Blend until smooth and creamy.
- Pour the smoothie mixture into a bowl.
- Top the smoothie bowl with granola, sliced almonds, and fresh berries.
- Enjoy this vitality-packed smoothie bowl that energizes your mornings and nourishes your body with essential nutrients.

1. Creamy Avocado and Smoked Salmon Toast

Ingredients:

- Two slices of whole-grain bread

- One ripe avocado
- One tablespoon of lemon juice
- Pinch of salt and black pepper
- Two oz smoked salmon
- Fresh dill or chives for garnish

Instructions:

1. Toast the slices of whole-grain bread to your desired level of crispiness.

2. Combine the ripe avocado with lemon juice, salt, and pepper in a bowl, mashing it together to create a creamy spread.

3. Spread the avocado mixture generously onto the toasted bread slices.

4. Top the avocado toast with smoked salmon and garnish with fresh dill or chives.

5. Indulge in this creamy and satisfying avocado toast that provides a delightful combination of healthy fats and protein.

6. Protein-Packed Banana Nut Pancakes

Ingredients:

- 1 cup oat flour (blended oats)
- One ripe banana, mashed
- 1/2 cup Greek yogurt
- Two eggs
- One tablespoon honey
- One teaspoon of baking powder
- Pinch of salt
- 1/4 cup chopped nuts (walnuts, almonds, or pecans)
- Coconut oil for cooking

Instructions:

1. Combine oat flour, mashed banana, Greek yogurt, eggs, honey, baking powder, and salt in a bowl. Blend until a smooth pancake batter is obtained.

2. Fold the chopped nuts into the batter.

3. Coat a non-stick pan with a thin layer of coconut oil and heat it over medium heat.

4. Pour some of the pancake batter into the hot pan, and cook it for two to three minutes on each side or until it turns a lovely golden brown.

5. Savor the protein-rich banana nut pancakes, topping them off with a drizzle of honey or maple syrup for a nourishing breakfast that invigorates your body with wholesome goodness.

2. High-Calorie Smoothie Bowl

Ingredients:

- One ripe banana
- 1 cup Greek yogurt
- 1/2 cup rolled oats
- 1/4 cup almond butter
- One tablespoon honey
- 1/2 cup mixed berries (strawberries, blueberries, or raspberries)
- One tablespoon of chia seeds
- 1/4 cup granola
- Sliced almonds and shredded coconut for topping

Instructions:

1. Combine the ripe banana, Greek yogurt, rolled oats, almond butter, and honey in a blender. Blend until smooth and creamy.

2. Pour the smoothie mixture into a bowl.

3. Top the smoothie bowl with mixed berries, chia seeds, granola, sliced almonds, and shredded coconut.

4. Enjoy this high-calorie and nutrient-rich breakfast to kickstart your day with energy and nourishment.

3. Avocado Toast Variations

Ingredients:

- Two slices of whole-grain bread
- One ripe avocado
- One tablespoon of lemon juice
- Pinch of salt and black pepper
- Optional toppings: sliced tomatoes, poached eggs, smoked salmon, or crumbled feta cheese

Instructions:

1. Toast the slices of whole-grain bread to your desired level of crispiness.

2. Mash the ripe avocado with lemon juice, salt, and black pepper in a bowl to make a smooth and creamy spread.

3. Spread the avocado mixture generously onto the toasted bread slices.

4. Customize your avocado toast by adding toppings like sliced tomatoes, poached eggs, smoked salmon, or crumbled feta cheese.

5. Each variation adds flavor and additional calories to your breakfast, making it a wholesome and satisfying choice.

4. Protein-Packed Pancakes

Ingredients:

- 1 cup oats (blended into fine flour)
- 1 ripe banana
- 1/2 cup Greek yogurt
- 2 eggs
- 1 teaspoon baking powder
- 1 teaspoon vanilla extract
- Pinch of salt
- Coconut oil for cooking

Instructions:

1. Process the oats using a blender or food processor until they reach a texture resembling flour.

2. Mash the ripe banana and whisk it with Greek yogurt, eggs, baking powder, vanilla extract, and salt until thoroughly blended.

3. Incorporate the oat flour into the wet ingredients, stirring until you achieve a smooth pancake batter.

4. Properly Heat a non-stick pan over medium heat and lightly grease it with a thin layer of coconut oil.

5. Pour a scoop of the pancake batter onto the hot pan, cooking for 2-3 minutes on each side until achieving a golden brown color.

6. Serve the protein-packed pancakes with a drizzle of honey, fresh berries, or a dollop of Greek yogurt to enhance the flavor and nutritional value.

Nourishing Lunches

These recipes are thoughtfully curated to provide the perfect blend of nutrients, flavor, and energy to keep you fueled and nourished throughout the day. They will satisfy your taste buds and contribute to your weight gain goals in a healthy and balanced manner.

1. Quinoa and Chickpea Power Salad

Ingredients:

- 1 cup cooked quinoa
- One can of chickpeas, drained and rinsed
- 1 cup cherry tomatoes, halved
- One cucumber, diced
- 1/4 cup chopped fresh parsley
- 1/4 cup crumbled feta cheese
- Two tablespoons extra-virgin olive oil
- One tablespoon of lemon juice
- Salt and pepper to taste

Instructions:

1. Combine cooked quinoa, chickpeas, cherry tomatoes, cucumber, and fresh parsley in a large mixing bowl.

2. Carefully Pour the olive oil and lemon juice on the salad, then mix and toss until the ingredients are thoroughly coated.

3. Season with salt and pepper to taste.

4. Top the salad with crumbled feta cheese for extra flavor and protein.

5. This nutrient-dense salad is a delicious and satisfying lunch option that will nourish your body with essential vitamins and minerals.

2. Mediterranean Grilled Chicken Grain Bowl

Ingredients:

- 1 cup cooked brown rice
- 4 oz grilled chicken breast, sliced
- 1/2 cup chopped cucumber
- 1/2 cup cherry tomatoes, halved
- 1/4 cup sliced Kalamata olives
- 1/4 cup crumbled feta cheese
- Two tablespoons of Greek yogurt dressing
- Fresh basil leaves for garnish

Instructions:

1. In a bowl, arrange the cooked brown rice as the base of the grain bowl.

2. Top with grilled chicken slices, chopped cucumber, cherry tomatoes, and Kalamata olives.

3. Sprinkle crumbled feta cheese over the ingredients.

4. Drizzle the Greek yogurt dressing over the grain bowl for added creaminess and flavor.

5. Garnish with fresh basil leaves for a touch of freshness, and serve this protein-packed lunch option.

3. Tuna Avocado Lettuce Wraps

Ingredients:

- One can of tuna, drained
- One ripe avocado, mashed
- One tablespoon of lemon juice
- Salt and pepper to taste
- Lettuce leaves for wrapping
- Sliced cucumbers and shredded carrots for topping

Instructions:

1. Mix the drained tuna with mashed avocado and lemon juice in a bowl.

2. Season with salt and pepper to taste.

3. Spoon the tuna avocado mixture onto lettuce leaves.

4. Top with sliced cucumbers and shredded carrots for added crunch and nutrition.

5. Roll up the lettuce leaves to create flavorful and satisfying wraps.

4. Hummus Veggie Wrap

Ingredients:

- Whole wheat tortilla
- 1/4 cup hummus
- Sliced bell peppers (red, yellow, and green)
- Sliced cucumbers
- Sliced carrots
- Spinach leaves

- Feta cheese (optional)

Instructions:

1. Lay the whole wheat tortilla flat and spread a generous layer of hummus over it.

2. Layer sliced bell peppers, cucumbers, carrots, and spinach leaves on the hummus.

3. Sprinkle feta cheese on the vegetables if desired.

4. Roll the tortilla tightly to form a delicious and nutrient-packed hummus veggie wrap.

5. Black Bean and Sweet Potato Buddha Bowl

Ingredients:

- 1 cup cooked quinoa
- One cup of black beans, cooked or canned, drained and rinsed
- One medium-sized sweet potato, roasted and diced
- 1/2 avocado, sliced
- Sliced red onions
- Two tablespoons of lime tahini dressing
- Fresh cilantro for garnish

Instructions:

1. Layer the cooked quinoa, black beans, roasted sweet potato, avocado slices, and sliced red onions in a bowl.

2. Drizzle the lime tahini dressing over the ingredients for a tangy and creamy touch.

3. Garnish with fresh cilantro for added flavor, and serve this wholesome and protein-rich Buddha bowl.

Nutrient-Loaded Dinners

Prepare to indulge in vibrant colors, tantalizing flavors, and various nourishing ingredients that satisfy and energize you. These nutrient-loaded dinners are thoughtfully crafted to nourish your body while providing a delightful dining experience.

1. Quinoa and Roasted Vegetable Buddha Bowl

Ingredients:

- 1 cup cooked quinoa
- 1 cup mixed roasted vegetables (such as sweet potatoes, bell peppers, and broccoli)
- 1/2 cup chickpeas, drained and rinsed
- 2 cups baby spinach or kale
- 1/4 avocado, sliced
- Two tablespoons hummus
- One tablespoon of olive oil
- One tablespoon of lemon juice
- Salt and pepper to taste

Instructions:

1. Combine the cooked quinoa, roasted vegetables, chickpeas, baby spinach, or kale in a large bowl.

2. Using a small bowl, mix the olive oil, lemon juice, salt, and pepper, whisking them together to create the dressing.

3. Drizzle the dressing over the quinoa and vegetable mixture and toss until well-coated.

4. Top the Buddha bowl with sliced avocado and a dollop of hummus for added creaminess and flavor.

5. Enjoy this nutrient-loaded dinner that balances healthy fats, lean proteins, and whole grains.

2. Salmon Stir-Fry with Sesame Ginger Sauce

Ingredients:

- One tablespoon of sesame oil
- One lb. salmon fillet, cut into bite-sized pieces
- Two cups mixed vegetables (such as bell peppers, snap peas, and carrots)
- Three tablespoons soy sauce (or tamari for a gluten-free option)
- One tablespoon honey
- One tablespoon of grated fresh ginger
- Two garlic cloves minced
- One tablespoon of sesame seeds
- Green onions, sliced (for garnish)
- Cooked brown rice (for serving)

Instructions:

1. Heat the sesame oil over medium-high heat in a large skillet or wok.

2. Add the salmon pieces and cook until browned and cooked through. Remove from the skillet and set aside.

3. In the same skillet, add the mixed vegetables and stir-fry until they are tender-crisp.

4. In a small bowl, whisk together the soy sauce, honey, grated ginger, and minced garlic to make the sauce.

5. Return the cooked salmon to the skillet and pour the sauce over the salmon and vegetables. Toss until well coated.

6. Sprinkle sesame seeds over the stir-fry for added crunch and flavor.

7. Serve the salmon stir-fry over cooked brown rice for a satisfying and protein-packed dinner.

3. Mediterranean Chickpea Pasta

Ingredients:

- Eight oz whole wheat pasta (or gluten-free pasta)
- One tablespoon of olive oil
- One onion, chopped
- Two garlic cloves minced
- One can of chickpeas, drained and rinsed
- 1 cup cherry tomatoes, halved
- 1/2 cup sliced black olives
- 1/4 cup chopped fresh basil
- 1/4 cup crumbled feta cheese (or dairy-free alternative)
- Lemon zest (from 1 lemon)
- Salt and pepper to taste

Instructions:

1. Prepare the pasta following the instructions on the package until it reaches an al dente consistency. Drain the pasta and set it aside.

2. Over a medium heat, heat the olive oil.

3. Add the chopped onion, minced garlic, and sauté until the onion is translucent.

4. Stir in the chickpeas, cherry tomatoes, and sliced black olives, and cook until heated.

5. Combine the cooked pasta with the chickpea mixture in the skillet, tossing until thoroughly combined.

6. Stir in the chopped fresh basil and crumbled feta cheese.

7. Season with lemon zest, salt, and pepper to taste.

8. Enjoy this Mediterranean-inspired chickpea pasta that provides a hearty and satisfying dinner.

4. Stuffed Bell Peppers with Quinoa and Black Beans

Ingredients:

- Four large bell peppers (any color), halved and seeds removed
- One cup of cooked quinoa
- One can of washed and drained black beans
- One cup of diced tomatoes
- 1 cup diced zucchini
- 1 cup diced red onion
- Fresh, frozen, or canned corn kernels totaling one cup
- Two cloves garlic, minced
- One teaspoon of ground cumin
- One teaspoon of chili powder
- Salt and pepper to taste

- 1/2 cup shredded cheddar cheese (or dairy-free alternative)

Instructions:

1. Set the oven temperature to 375°F (190°C).

2. In a large skillet, sauté the diced red onion and minced garlic until the onion is translucent.

3. Add the diced tomatoes, zucchini, and corn kernels to the skillet and cook until the vegetables are tender.

4. Stir in the cooked quinoa and black beans, and season with ground cumin, chili powder, salt, and pepper.

5. Arrange the halved bell peppers in a baking dish and stuff them with the quinoa and black bean mixture.

6. Sprinkle shredded cheddar cheese over the stuffed bell peppers.

7. When the bell peppers are soft, and the cheese is melted, cover the baking dish using aluminum foil and bake it in the oven for 25 to 30 minutes.

8. Serve the stuffed bell peppers as a hearty vegetable-based main, perfect for a satisfying dinner.

5. Baked Sweet Potato with Chickpea and Avocado Salsa

Ingredients:

- Two large sweet potatoes
- One can of chickpeas, drained and rinsed
- One avocado, diced
- 1 cup cherry tomatoes, halved

- 1/4 cup chopped fresh cilantro
- One lime, juiced
- One tablespoon of olive oil
- Salt and pepper to taste

Instructions:

1. Set the oven's temperature to 400°F (200°C).

2. Put the sweet potatoes on a baking pan and pierce them with a fork.

3. Bake the sweet potatoes in the oven for 40-45 minutes or until tender.

4. Mix the chickpeas, diced avocado, cherry tomatoes, fresh cilantro, lime juice, extra virgin olive oil, salt, and pepper together in a bowl to make the salsa.

5. Once the sweet potatoes are baked, cut them open and stuff them with chickpea and avocado salsa.

6. Enjoy this nutrient-loaded dinner featuring the natural sweetness of baked sweet potatoes and the fresh flavors of chickpea and avocado salsa.

These nutrient-loaded recipes cater to the desire for satisfying and wholesome meals by incorporating healthy fats, lean proteins, and whole grains. They provide a range of options to please every palate while supporting the goal of gaining weight in a healthy and balanced way. Enjoy these nutrient-packed dinners and embrace the delicious and nourishing flavors they offer.

SECTION 3: RECIPES FOR WEIGHT LOSS

In the pursuit of achieving the ideal body or rapid weight loss, the minds of many individuals have been preoccupied. Whether driven by health concerns or aesthetic aspirations, they all share a common goal - shedding those extra pounds quickly and effectively.

However, the key to successful weight loss lies in the program and choosing the right one that suits individual needs. Understanding this crucial aspect ensures an efficient and sustainable weight loss journey. Fortunately, specific recipes have proven highly effective in aiding rapid weight loss while promoting overall well-being.

This section delves into the culinary secrets that can help accelerate weight loss. These recipes have been thoughtfully curated, offering a balanced and nourishing approach to shedding those unwanted pounds. So, let's delve into these essential and health-conscious recipes that can pave the way to achieving your weight loss goals.

1. Quinoa and Vegetable Stir-Fry

Ingredients:

- 1 cup cooked quinoa
- One tablespoon of olive oil
- One cup of mixed vegetables (such as bell peppers, broccoli, and carrots)
- 1/2 cup edamame (shelled)
- Two tablespoons of low-sodium soy sauce
- One tablespoon of sesame oil
- One tablespoon of rice vinegar
- One teaspoon of grated ginger

- One clove of garlic, minced
- One tablespoon of sesame seeds
- Fresh cilantro for garnish

Instructions:

1. Heat the olive oil in a sizable skillet or wok over medium-high heat.

2. Stir-fry the mixed vegetables and edamame for 3 to 4 minutes or until soft but crunchy.

3. To make the sauce, combine the soy sauce, sesame oil, rice vinegar, grated ginger, and minced garlic in a small bowl.

4. Add cooked quinoa to the skillet, followed by the sauce. Toss everything together until well coated.

5. Sprinkle sesame seeds over the stir-fry and garnish with fresh cilantro.

6. Serve immediately, promoting mindful eating and savoring each nutritious bite.

2. Mediterranean Stuffed Bell Peppers

Ingredients:

- Four large bell peppers (any color), halved and seeds removed
- 1 cup cooked brown rice
- One can (15 oz) chickpeas, drained and rinsed
- 1 cup diced tomatoes
- 1/2 cup chopped cucumber
- 1/4 cup chopped red onion
- 1/4 cup crumbled feta cheese (or dairy-free alternative)
- Two tablespoons chopped fresh parsley

- One tablespoon of lemon juice
- One tablespoon of olive oil
- Pepper and salt as desired

Instructions:

1. Prepare a baking dish and preheat the oven to 375°F (190°C).

2. Mix cooked brown rice, chickpeas, diced tomatoes, chopped cucumber, chopped red onion, and crumbled feta cheese in a large bowl.

3. To create the dressing, whisk the lemon juice together with olive oil, salt, and pepper in a small bowl.

4. Drizzle the dressing over the rice mixture and toss until well combined.

5. Stuff each bell pepper half with the Mediterranean mixture.

6. Arrange the stuffed bell peppers in the baking dish, then cover them with foil and bake for 20-25 minutes until the peppers become tender.

7. Serve the Mediterranean stuffed bell peppers, emphasizing portion control and enjoying a balanced and flavorful meal.

3. Green Goddess Buddha Bowl

Ingredients:

- 1 cup cooked quinoa
- 1 cup kale or spinach leaves
- 1/2 cup cooked chickpeas
- 1/2 avocado, sliced
- 1/4 cup sliced cucumber
- 1/4 cup shredded carrots

- Two tablespoons hummus
- Two tablespoons lemon-tahini dressing
- Fresh dill for garnish

Instructions:

1. In a serving bowl, arrange cooked quinoa, kale or spinach leaves, and cooked chickpeas.

2. Add sliced avocado, sliced cucumber, and shredded carrots to the bowl.

3. Drizzle hummus and lemon-tahini dressing over the ingredients.

4. Garnish with fresh dill.

5. Toss the ingredients together before eating, ensuring mindful consumption of each nutrient-packed element.

4. Baked Salmon with Asparagus and Lemon

Ingredients:

- Four salmon fillets
- One bunch of asparagus, trimmed
- One lemon, sliced
- Two tablespoons of olive oil
- Two cloves garlic, minced
- One teaspoon of dried thyme
- Salt and pepper to taste

Instructions:

1. To begin, set the oven to a temperature of 400°F (200°C) and arrange a baking sheet using parchment paper.

2. Place the salmon fillets and trimmed asparagus on the baking sheet.

3. In a small bowl, mix together the olive oil, minced garlic, dried thyme, salt, and pepper until thoroughly blended.

4. Make sure the salmon and asparagus are well covered by drizzling the olive oil mixture over them.

5. Arrange lemon slices on top of the salmon and asparagus.

6. Bake the salmon and asparagus in the oven for 12 -15 minutes, depending on how done you want your salmon.

7. Serve the baked salmon and asparagus, promoting portion control and balanced nutrition.

5. Berry and Chia Seed Smoothie

Ingredients:

- 1 cup mixed berries (strawberries, blueberries, raspberries)
- One ripe banana
- One tablespoon of chia seeds
- 1 cup unsweetened almond milk (or any preferred milk)
- One tablespoon honey (optional for added sweetness)
- Ice cubes (optional for a chilled smoothie)

Instructions:

1. In a blender, combine mixed berries, ripe bananas, chia seeds, almond milk, and honey (if using).

2. Blend until smooth and creamy.

3. If desired, add ice cubes and blend again for a chilled smoothie.

4. Pour the berry and chia seed smoothie into a glass, practicing mindful eating by savoring the delicious and nutritious flavors.

Wholesome Breakfasts

Maintaining a healthy diet with a nourishing breakfast daily is crucial to achieving and preserving a regular and wholesome body weight. As previously mentioned, the benefits of starting your day with a proper breakfast extend beyond just satisfying hunger; it is also closely linked to weight control. By incorporating the following recipes into your daily routine, you can support your weight loss goals while enjoying delicious and nutritious morning meals.

1. Green Protein Smoothie

Ingredients:

- One cup of spinach or kale leaves
- 1/2 cucumber, peeled and chopped
- 1/2 avocado
- 1/2 cup almond milk without sugar (or any other favorite milk)
- One tablespoon of chia seeds
- One tablespoon of almond butter
- 1/2 teaspoon honey (optional for added sweetness)
- Ice cubes (optional for a chilled smoothie)

Instructions:

1. In a blender, combine spinach or kale leaves, chopped cucumber, avocado, almond milk, chia seeds, almond butter, and honey (if using).

2. Blend until smooth and creamy.

3. If desired, add ice cubes and blend again for a refreshing and low-calorie green protein smoothie.

4. Transfer the smoothie into a glass and begin your day with a nourishing and weight-loss-friendly breakfast.

2. Berry Overnight Oats

Ingredients:

- 1/2 cup rolled oats
- One cup of unsweetened almond milk (or your preferred choice of milk).
- A quarter cup of Greek yogurt (or a dairy-free alternative).
- 1/2 cup mixed berries (strawberries, blueberries, raspberries)
- A single tablespoon of chia seeds.
- If preferred, add a spoonful of honey or maple syrup for sweetness.
- One tablespoon of sliced almonds or chopped walnuts (optional, for crunch)

Instructions:

1. In a Mason jar or airtight container, combine rolled oats, almond milk, Greek yogurt, mixed berries, and chia seeds.

2. Stir everything together until well-mixed.

3. If desired, drizzle honey or maple syrup for added sweetness.

4. Cover the container and refrigerate overnight.

5. In the morning, stir the oats well and sprinkle sliced almonds or chopped walnuts for a delightful and nutritious crunch.

6. Enjoy the convenience and wholesomeness of this weight-loss-friendly berry overnight oats.

3. Veggie-Packed Egg White Omelette

Ingredients:

- Four egg whites cup and a half of finely diced, any color bell peppers.
- 1/4 cup diced tomatoes
- 1/4 cup sliced mushrooms
- 1/4 cup chopped spinach
- One tablespoon of chopped fresh basil or parsley
- Salt and pepper to taste
- One teaspoon of olive oil

Instructions:

1. In a dish, whisk the egg whites until they are foamy.

2. In a non-stick skillet, warm up the olive oil over medium heat.

3. Add chopped bell peppers, diced tomatoes, sliced mushrooms, and chopped spinach to the skillet. Sauté until vegetables are tender.

4. Pour the whisked egg whites over the sautéed vegetables in the skillet.

5. Cook the omelet until the edges are set and the center is slightly runny.

6. Carefully fold the omelet in half and cook for another minute until fully set.

7. Sprinkle chopped fresh basil or parsley, salt, and pepper over the omelet for added flavor.

8. Serve this veggie-packed egg white omelet, providing a protein-rich and nutritious breakfast to fuel your day.

4. Avocado Toast with Poached Egg

Ingredients:

- Two slices of whole-grain bread (or gluten-free bread)
- One ripe avocado, mashed
- Two poached eggs
- One tablespoon of chopped fresh cilantro
- Salt and pepper to taste
- Crushed red pepper flakes (optional for added spice)

Instructions:

1. Toast the whole-grain bread slices until golden brown.

2. Spread the mashed avocado evenly on the toasted bread slices.

3. Top each avocado toast with a poached egg.

4. Sprinkle chopped fresh cilantro, salt, and pepper over the poached eggs.

5. For a spicy kick, add some crushed red pepper flakes.

6. Savor this avocado toast's creamy and nutritious goodness with poached egg, perfect for a satisfying and weight-loss-friendly breakfast.

5. Chia Seed Pudding with Fresh Fruit

Ingredients:

- 1/4 cup chia seeds
- A cup of almond milk without sugar (or your favorite milk)
- One teaspoon of honey or maple syrup (optional for added sweetness)
- 1/2 cup of assorted fresh fruit (such as thinly sliced strawberries, blueberries, or kiwis)
- One tablespoon of sliced almonds or chopped walnuts (optional, for crunch)

Instructions:

1. In a bowl, mix chia seeds and almond milk until well combined.

2. If desired, add honey or maple syrup for added sweetness.

3. Place a cover over the bowl and refrigerate for 3-4 hours or overnight, enabling the chia seeds to thicken.

4. In the morning, give the chia seed pudding a good stir.

5. Layer the chia seed pudding with mixed fresh fruit in a glass or bowl.

6. Top with sliced almonds or chopped walnuts for a delightful crunch and added nutrients.

7. Enjoy this refreshing and low-calorie chia seed pudding with fresh fruit as a perfect start to your day.

With these wholesome breakfast recipes, you have various nutritious options to support your weight loss goals.

Light and Flavorful Lunches

Suppose you've been looking for light and flavorful recipe ideas that won't compromise on flavor or leave you unsatisfied. In that case, you've arrived at a culinary oasis designed to elevate your dining experience. The quest for weight loss often conjures images of bland, uninspiring meals that dampen your enthusiasm for healthy eating. But fear not for these mouthwatering lunch recipes that prove you can achieve your wellness goals without sacrificing the joy of food.

1. Summer Chickpea Salad

Ingredients

- One can (15 oz) of washed and drained chickpeas
- One cup of cherry tomatoes, halved
- One cup of diced cumber
- One small red onion, thinly sliced
- 1/4 cup chopped fresh parsley
- 1/4 cup crumbled feta cheese
- Two tablespoons extra-virgin olive oil
- Two tablespoons of lemon juice
- Salt and pepper to taste

Instructions:

1. In a large bowl, combine chickpeas, cherry tomatoes, cucumber, red onion, and parsley.

2. Combine the ingredients for the dressing—olive oil, lemon juice, salt, and pepper—in a small dish.

3. Add the salad to the dressing and gently mix to incorporate.

4. Sprinkle the crumbled feta cheese on top.

5. Serve chilled, and enjoy this refreshing and protein-packed salad.

2. Butternut Squash and Carrot Soup

Ingredients:

- One medium butternut squash, diced after being skinned and seeded
- Three large carrots, peeled and chopped
- One small onion, chopped
- Two cloves garlic, minced
- Four cups vegetable broth
- One teaspoon of ground cumin
- 1/2 teaspoon ground ginger
- Salt and pepper to taste
- One tablespoon of olive oil
- Fresh cilantro or parsley for garnish

Instructions:

1. In a big saucepan set over medium heat, warm the olive oil. Onion and garlic should be added and sautéed until transparent.

2. Add the butternut squash, carrots, vegetable broth, cumin, ginger, salt, and pepper to the saucepan.

3. Heat the mixture to a boil, then lower the heat and simmer it for 20 to 25 minutes or until the veggies are fork-tender.

4. Using an immersion or regular blender, puree the soup until smooth and creamy.

5. Adjust seasoning if needed.

6. Serve the soup hot, garnished with fresh cilantro or parsley.

3. Greek Chicken Wrap with Tzatziki Sauce

Ingredients:

- Two whole wheat tortillas or wraps
- One cup of cooked chicken breast, sliced
- 1/2 cup cherry tomatoes, halved
- 1/4 cup sliced cucumber
- 1/4 cup sliced red onion
- Two tablespoons of crumbled feta cheese
- Fresh lettuce leaves

For Tzatziki Sauce:

- 1/2 cup Greek yogurt
- 1/4 cup grated cucumber, squeezed to remove excess water
- One clove of garlic, minced
- One tablespoon of lemon juice
- One tablespoon of chopped fresh dill
- Salt and pepper to taste

Instructions:

1. Combine all the Tzatziki sauce ingredients in a small dish and leave aside.

2. Lay the whole wheat tortillas or wraps on a clean surface.

3. On each wrap, spread a generous amount of Tzatziki sauce in the center.

4. Top with sliced chicken, cherry tomatoes, cucumber, red onion, feta cheese, and fresh lettuce leaves.

5. Fold in the sides of the wrap and roll it tightly.

6. Slice each wrap in half and serve immediately.

4. Quinoa Avocado Salad with Lemon-Herb Dressing

Ingredients:

- One cup of cooked quinoa
- One ripe avocado, diced
- One cup of cherry tomatoes, halved
- 1/2 cucumber, diced
- 1/4 cup red onion, finely chopped
- 1/4 cup fresh cilantro, chopped
- Two tablespoons of fresh mint, chopped
- Two tablespoons of extra-virgin olive oil
- Juice of 1 lemon
- One garlic clove, minced
- Salt and pepper to taste

Instructions:

1. Place the cooked quinoa, diced avocado, cherry tomatoes, cucumber, red onion, fresh cilantro, and mint in a large mixing bowl.

2. To prepare the lemon-herb dressing, combine the extra virgin olive oil, lemon juice, garlic that has been minced, salt, and pepper in a separate small bowl.

3. After adding the dressing, gently toss the quinoa and avocado mixture to cover everything.

4. Allow the salad 5 minutes to let the flavors meld together.

5. Serve the quinoa avocado salad immediately, or refrigerate for later. It can be enjoyed independently or as a grilled chicken or fish dish.

5: Grilled Chicken and Vegetable Wrap

Ingredients:

- Two whole wheat tortillas
- Two boneless, skinless chicken breasts
- One zucchini, sliced lengthwise
- One red bell pepper, sliced
- One tablespoon of olive oil
- One teaspoon paprika
- 1/2 teaspoon garlic powder
- Salt and pepper to taste
- 1/4 cup hummus
- 1/4 cup baby spinach leaves
- 1/4 cup shredded carrots
- 1/4 cup sliced cucumber

Instructions:

1. Preheat your grill or grill pan over medium-high heat.

2. Sprinkle salt, pepper, paprika, garlic powder, and olive oil on the chicken breasts.

3. Grill the chicken breasts for 6-7 minutes per side or until they reach an internal temperature of 165°F (74°C). Remove from the grill and let them rest for a few minutes before slicing.

4. While the chicken grills, brush the zucchini and red bell pepper slices with olive oil and season with salt and pepper.

5. Grill the vegetables for 2-3 minutes per side until they are slightly charred and tender.

6. Warm the whole wheat tortillas on the grill for 30 seconds on each side.

7. To assemble the wrap, spread two tablespoons of hummus onto each tortilla.

8. Place sliced grilled chicken, zucchini, and red bell pepper onto the center of each tortilla.

9. Top with baby spinach leaves, shredded carrots, and sliced cucumber.

10. Roll up the tortilla tightly, tucking in the sides as you go.

11. Cut the wraps in half diagonally and serve right away, or wrap them in foil for a lunch that can be taken with you.

These delicious and nutritious lunch dishes can sate your appetite while helping you stick to your weight loss objectives.

Enjoy the vibrant flavors and ingredients, knowing you're nourishing your body while indulging in delicious meals! Bon appétit!

Balanced Dinners

When planning dinner with weight loss in mind, try to choose a healthy, balanced meal that supports your wellness objectives and pleases your palate.

As the sun sets, it's the perfect time to savor a fulfilling dinner that nourishes your body and satisfies your soul. Finding the right balance between flavor, texture, and nutritional content is essential, and that's where these balanced recipes for weight loss come to the rescue.

1. Baked Lemon Herb Salmon with Quinoa and Steamed Broccoli

Ingredients:

- Two salmon fillets
- Two tablespoons of olive oil
- Juice of 1 lemon
- One teaspoon of dried oregano
- One teaspoon of dried thyme
- Salt and pepper to taste
- 1 cup cooked quinoa
- Steamed broccoli florets

Instructions:

1. Set the oven's temperature to 400°F (200°C).

2. Combine olive oil, lemon juice, dried thyme, dried oregano, and salt & pepper in a small dish.

3. Place the salmon fillets on a baking sheet lined with parchment paper.

4. Brush the salmon with the lemon herb mixture, coating both sides.

5. Bake the salmon for 12-15 minutes or until it's cooked and flakes easily with a fork.

6. Serve the baked lemon herb salmon over a bed of cooked quinoa and steamed broccoli.

2. Lentil and Vegetable Stir-Fry

Ingredients:

- One cup of cooked lentils
- One tablespoon of sesame oil
- One small onion, thinly sliced
- One red bell pepper, thinly sliced
- 1 cup broccoli florets
- 1 cup sliced mushrooms
- Two tablespoons of low-sodium soy sauce
- One tablespoon of rice vinegar
- One teaspoon grated ginger
- Two cloves garlic, minced
- Sesame seeds (optional)
- Cooked brown rice (to serve)

Instructions:

1. In a large skillet or wok, warm the sesame oil over medium heat.

2. Add sliced onion, red bell pepper, broccoli, and mushrooms. Stir-fry for 3-4 minutes until vegetables are tender-crisp.

3. Stir in cooked lentils and cook for an additional 2 minutes.

4. Mix soy sauce, rice vinegar, chopped garlic, and grated ginger in a small bowl.

5. Pour the sauce over the stir-fry and toss everything together until well-coated.

6. Sprinkle with sesame seeds (if using) and serve over cooked brown rice.

3. Shrimp and Veggie Stir-Fry with Cauliflower Rice

Ingredients:

- One pound of shrimp, peeled and deveined
- One tablespoon of olive oil
- One red bell pepper, thinly sliced
- One cup sliced carrots
- One cup snap peas
- Two cups cauliflower rice (store-bought or homemade)
- Two tablespoons of low-sodium soy sauce
- One tablespoon of hoisin sauce
- One teaspoon of sesame oil
- Two green onions, sliced (for garnish)

Instructions:

1. In a big wok or saucepan, heat the olive oil over medium-high heat.

2. Add shrimp and stir-fry until pink and cooked through. Remove from the skillet and set aside.

3. In the same skillet, add sliced red bell pepper, sliced carrots, and snap peas. Stir-fry for 3-4 minutes until vegetables are tender-crisp.

4. Stir constantly for 2 minutes while cooking the cauliflower rice in the skillet.

5. Mix soy sauce, hoisin sauce, and sesame oil in a small bowl.

6. Pour the sauce over the stir-fry and toss everything together until well-coated.

7. Add the cooked shrimp back to the skillet and toss to combine.

8. Garnish with sliced green onions before serving.

4. Baked Stuffed Portobello Mushrooms

Ingredients:

- Four large Portobello mushroom stems removed
- One tablespoon of olive oil
- One small onion, finely chopped
- Two cloves garlic, minced
- One cup of chopped spinach
- One cup of diced tomatoes (canned or fresh)
- 1/2 cup cooked quinoa
- 1/4 cup grated Parmesan cheese (optional)
- Salt and pepper to taste
- Fresh basil leaves (for garnish)

Instructions:

1. Regulate the oven's temperature to 375°F (190°C).

2. Place the Portobello mushrooms on a baking sheet, gill-side up.

3. Heat the olive oil to medium-high heat. Sauté the chopped onion and minced garlic until softened.

4. Stir in chopped spinach and diced tomatoes, cook until the spinach is wilted.

5. After turning off the heat, add the cooked quinoa and, if desired, some grated Parmesan cheese to the pan.

6. Add pepper and salt to taste when preparing the mixture.

7. Stuff each Portobello mushroom with the quinoa and vegetable mixture.

8. Bake for 15 to 20 minutes or until the filling is hot and the mushrooms are soft.

9. Garnish with fresh basil leaves before serving.

5. Veggie and Tofu Stir-Fry with Brown Rice

Ingredients:

- One cup of cubed tofu
- Two tablespoons of low-sodium soy sauce
- One tablespoon of cornstarch
- One tablespoon of sesame oil
- One tablespoon of olive oil
- One small onion, thinly sliced
- One cup of sliced bell peppers (any color)
- One cup of sliced carrots

- One cup of sliced snap peas
- Two cups of cooked brown rice

Instructions:

1. In a bowl, toss cubed tofu with low-sodium soy sauce and cornstarch until coated.

2. Heat the sesame and olive oils over medium-high heat.

3. Add the marinated tofu to the skillet and stir-fry until golden and crispy. Remove from the skillet and set aside.

4. In the same skillet, add sliced onion, bell peppers, carrots, and snap peas. Stir-fry for 3-4 minutes until vegetables are tender-crisp.

5. Add the cooked tofu back to the skillet and toss to combine.

6. Serve the veggie and tofu stir-fry over a bed of cooked brown rice.

6. Mediterranean Chickpea Salad

Ingredients:

- Two cups of cooked chickpeas (canned or soaked and cooked)
- A cup of diced cucumber
- One cup of halved cherry tomatoes
- 1/2 cup diced red onion
- 1/4 cup pitted Kalamata olives, halved
- 1/4 cup crumbled feta cheese (optional)
- Two tablespoons extra-virgin olive oil
- Juice of 1 lemon
- One teaspoon of dried oregano

- Salt and pepper to taste
- Fresh parsley leaves (for garnish)

Instructions:

1. In a sized mixing bowl, blend together cooked chickpeas, diced cucumber, halved cherry tomatoes, diced red onion, and halved Kalamata olives.

2. If using feta cheese, add it to the bowl.

3. Using a separate small bowl, whisk together extra-virgin olive oil, lemon juice, dried oregano, salt, and pepper to make the dressing.

4. After adding the dressing, gently mix the chickpea salad to uniformly distribute the ingredients.

5. Allow the salad a few minutes to let the flavors meld together.6. Before serving, garnish with fresh parsley leaves.

Note: Consuming your dinner at least 2-3 hours before bedtime is recommended. This gives your body enough time to digest the food and avoid discomfort while sleeping.

SECTION 4: TIPS FOR SUCCESS AND SUSTAINABILITY

Achieving your target weight is a journey that varies from person to person. There is no one-size-fits-all approach, so these tips empower you with the knowledge and tools to customize your path according to your unique needs, lifestyle, and preferences. By embracing these suggestions, you can embark on a personalized weight management journey that aligns perfectly with your goals.

Tips On How To Achieve Weight Gain Or Weight Loss Goals In a Sustainable Manner

Whether you aim to gain weight healthily or lose unwanted pounds, sustainably achieving your goals is essential for long-term success. Crash diets and extreme approaches may yield quick results, but they often lead to rebound weight gain or other health issues. Instead, adopting a balanced and sustainable approach is key to reaching your desired weight and maintaining it in the long run.

Below are some practical tips to assist you in achieving your weight gain or weight loss objectives sustainably and healthily.

1. Set Realistic Goals

The first step towards achieving sustainable weight gain or weight loss is setting realistic and achievable goals. Be honest with yourself about your starting point and your desired outcome. Set incremental, attainable goals, and celebrate your progress along the way. Unrealistic expectations can lead to frustration and discouragement, making staying committed to your journey harder.

2. Understand Your Caloric Needs

Understanding your daily caloric needs to gain or lose weight is essential. Use online calculators or seek advice from a healthcare professional to ascertain your basal metabolic rate (BMR) and consider your activity level to estimate your Total Daily Energy Expenditure (TDEE). Knowing your caloric needs will help you create an appropriate meal plan and make necessary adjustments to support your weight goals.

3. Focus on Nutrient-Dense Foods

Whether you want to gain or lose weight, prioritizing nutrient-dense foods is crucial. Focusing on nutrient-dense foods, abundant in vital vitamins, minerals, and other advantageous compounds while being relatively lower in calories is crucial for optimizing your body's fuel and promoting overall well-being. To achieve this, include a diverse array of fruits, vegetables, whole grains, lean meats, and healthy fats in your daily diet.

4. Mindful Eating

Practicing mindful eating is beneficial for both weight gain and weight loss goals. Remember your hunger and fullness cues, and avoid distractions while eating. Engage in mindful eating by chewing your food thoroughly and relishing each bite, enabling your body to recognize satisfaction. This practice can prevent overeating and foster a positive relationship with food.

5. Keep a Food Journal

Maintaining a food journal can be valuable in monitoring your food intake and recognizing eating patterns. Document every item you eat and drink, portion sizes, and consumption time. This practice promotes accountability, allows you to identify areas for improvement, and facilitates necessary adjustments to align with your weight goals.

6. Regular Physical Activity

Regular physical exercise is essential for general health and achieving your weight goals, whether you want to gain or reduce weight.

Discover physical activities you enjoy, such as walking, jogging, swimming, or dancing, to ensure a sustainable and enjoyable fitness regimen. Engaging in regular exercise not only burns calories but also boosts metabolism, improves mood, and enhances overall well-being.

7. Strength Training for Weight Gain

Incorporating strength training exercises is beneficial for those looking to gain weight healthily. Strength training in your exercise program is helpful for muscle mass increase, which leads to healthy weight gain.

Prioritize compound exercises such as squats, deadlifts, and bench presses, and complement your efforts with a balanced diet that supports muscle growth.

8. Portion Control for Weight Loss

For weight loss goals, portion control is essential. Be mindful of portion sizes and avoid oversized servings, especially high-calorie foods. Opt for smaller plates to create the illusion of satisfaction with smaller portions, effectively tricking your brain. Achieving sustainable weight loss depends on balancing your caloric intake and physical activity levels.

9. Stay Hydrated

Proper hydration is vital for both weight gain and weight loss journeys. Drinking enough water not only aids digestion and nutrient absorption but also helps control hunger and prevent overeating. Don't forget to stay hydrated throughout the day and avoid confusing thirst with hunger.

10. Seek Support

Whether you aim to gain or lose weight, seeking support can be incredibly beneficial. Join a community or find a weight loss or weight gain buddy to share experiences, celebrate successes, and provide motivation during challenging times. Furthermore, it is important to seek the advice of a certified dietician or healthcare expert to establish a personalized plan that aligns with your specific requirements and goals.

Achieving weight gain or weight loss goals sustainably requires commitment, patience, and a balanced approach. Remember that sustainable weight management is not about quick fixes but about making positive lifestyle changes you can maintain in the long run. Embrace the process, celebrate your progress, and enjoy the transformative power of sustainable weight gain or weight loss.

The Importance Of Incorporating Exercise And Staying Hydrated.

In pursuing a healthy and balanced lifestyle, two fundamental pillars are crucial: regular exercise and proper hydration. Both exercise and staying hydrated are integral in supporting overall well-being, promoting optimal physical and mental health, and achieving fitness goals.

Exercise

Incorporating regular physical activity into your lifestyle is fundamental to maintaining overall health and well-being. Whether it involves a structured workout routine or participating in daily activities that keep your body in motion, exercise offers many benefits that profoundly impact both the body and mind.

1. Weight Management: Exercise is critical to weight management by burning calories and increasing metabolism. Combining regular physical activity with a balanced diet can aid in weight loss or maintenance.

2. Muscle Strength and Endurance: Engaging in resistance training or strength-building exercises helps to increase muscle mass and improve muscular endurance. Strong muscles support proper posture, reduce the risk of injuries, and enhance overall physical performance.

3. Cardiovascular Health: Aerobic exercises, such as running, cycling, and swimming, improve cardiovascular health by strengthening the heart and enhancing blood circulation. Regular cardio workouts reduce the risk of heart disease, high blood pressure, and stroke.

4. Bone Health: Weight-bearing exercises like walking or dancing benefit bone health. They help maintain bone density, reduce the risk of osteoporosis, and support joint health.

5. Mental Well-being: Exercise profoundly impacts mental health, promoting the release of endorphins, also known as "feel-good" hormones. Regular physical activity reduces stress, anxiety, and symptoms of depression, leading to improved mood and emotional well-being.

6. Enhanced Energy and Stamina: Regular exercise boosts energy levels and stamina. Physical activity improves oxygen circulation and nutrient delivery to tissues, making daily tasks easier.

Hydration

Proper hydration is essential for maintaining optimal body functions and supporting overall health. Water is a vital nutrient that our bodies require for various physiological processes. Staying hydrated offers numerous benefits and is crucial for our well-being.

1. Regulation of Body Temperature: Water helps regulate body temperature by releasing heat through sweat during physical activity or in hot environments. Proper hydration prevents overheating and helps maintain a stable body temperature.

2. Digestion and Nutrient Absorption: Hydration is pivotal in digestion, as it aids in breaking down food and facilitates the efficient absorption of nutrients within the intestines. Staying hydrated ensures proper digestion and enhances the body's ability to utilize essential nutrients effectively.

3. Removal of Toxins: Sufficient hydration supports kidney function by assisting in the filtration of waste and toxins from the body via urine. Additionally, it aids in eliminating waste products, contributing to the overall detoxification process.

4. Joint and Tissue Health: Water is a lubricant for joints, helping reduce friction and preventing joint pain or stiffness. Proper hydration also supports the health and flexibility of muscles and connective tissues.

5. Cognitive Function: Dehydration can negatively impact cognitive function, decreasing alertness, concentration, and memory. Staying hydrated enhances cognitive performance and mental clarity.

6. Skin Health: Proper hydration promotes healthy and radiant skin by maintaining elasticity and preventing dryness. It helps flush out toxins, reducing the risk of skin problems and supporting a youthful appearance.

To fully reap the benefits of exercise and hydration, it is essential to incorporate them into our daily routines. So, let's take that extra step, drink that glass of water, and move our bodies to experience the transformative power of exercise and hydration on our journey toward well-being and vitality.

Conclusion

The significance of quick recipes tailored to specific weight gain and weight loss goals cannot be overstated. We recognize the value of optimizing time while focusing on healthy eating. These culinary solutions offer a pragmatic approach to achieving our desired weight outcomes without compromising nutrition or flavor.

We extend an encouraging call to embark on this culinary journey enthusiastically and creatively. Embrace the joy of experimenting with diverse ingredients, flavors, and cooking techniques. Customize these quick recipes to suit your tastes and dietary requirements, making each meal a delightful expression of your culinary prowess.

As we savor the fruits of our culinary endeavors, let us not lose sight of the broader picture—a healthy lifestyle that extends beyond the confines of the kitchen. Balanced nutrition, mindful eating, and regular exercise are timeless principles that underpin our overall well-being, irrespective of our weight objectives.

Balanced nutrition provides the essential building blocks for robust physical health and cognitive function. By incorporating a wide range of nutrient-rich foods into our diets, we nourish our bodies and lay the groundwork for vitality and longevity. Mindful eating, like the art of precision seasoning, adds depth and mindfulness to our dining experiences. By savoring each bite, recognizing hunger cues, and fostering a positive relationship with food, we establish a harmonious and sustainable approach to eating.

Like a steadfast sous-chef, regular exercise supports our weight goals while offering additional benefits. Physical activity elevates our mood, strengthens our bodies, and improves overall health and confidence.

Quick recipes tailored to weight gain and weight loss goals provide a pragmatic and effective path to culinary satisfaction and physical well-being. As we navigate our busy lives, remember that our culinary choices are integral to a holistic and healthy lifestyle.

So, let's seize the opportunities presented by these quick and wholesome recipes. Embrace the pleasure of culinary creativity, mindful eating, and regular exercise. With each meal, we savor the promise of a vibrant life of purpose, joy, and dedication to our long-term health and wellness. Bon appétit to a life well lived!